# Of Cautious Steps

## Darren Black

LILY POETRY REVIEW BOOKS

Copyright © 2024 by Darren Black
Published by Lily Poetry Review Books
223 Winter Street
Whitman, MA 02382

https://lilypoetryreview.blog/

ISBN: 978-1-957755-43-4

All rights reserved. Published in the United States by Lily Poetry Review Books. Library of Congress Control Number: 2024945195

Cover and author photos: Debi Milligan

*For Loretta, my mom, in memory.*

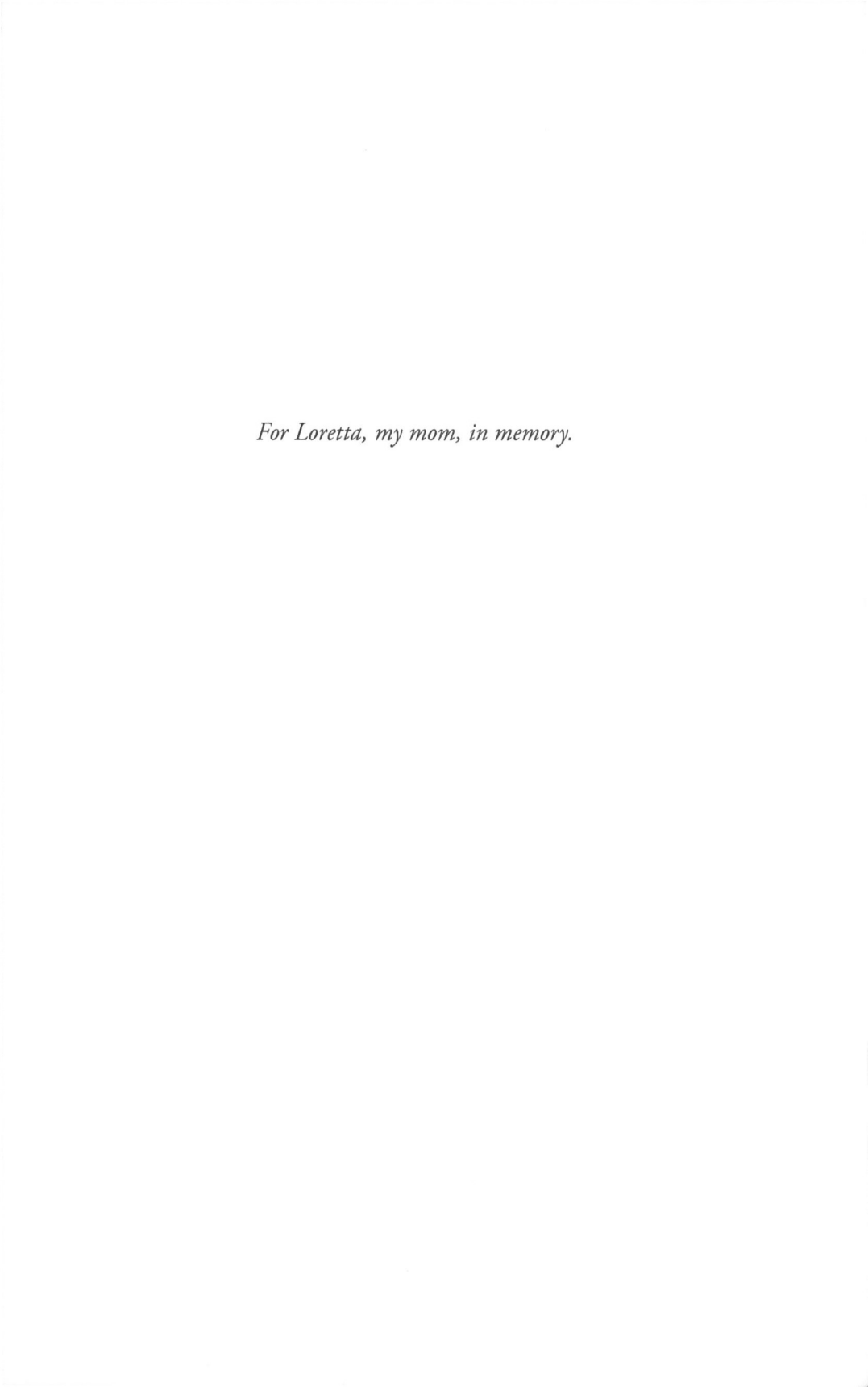

Scan code to hear Darren Black
read from *Of Cautious Steps*

## Table of Contents

1. While Waiting for the Ophthalmologist's Prognosis
2. Istanbul Busker
3. A Single Damn Word Never Finished
4. Mainstream Test Case 1973
5. Eminent Domain
6. SM Origin Story
7. Slow Night
8. Drinking Alone
9. How to Love a Mermaid
10. Night Muse Gathers More Pulp for the Cosmic Pile
11. Snow Event
12. Winter Ground
13. Quarantine Window
14. Glottal Stops
16. Postcolonial Island Hopping
18. Lady Liberty Begins to Fidget
19. Public Art
20. The Propellers
21. At the Canyon
23. The Day I Deleted My Fitness App
24. A Vision Therapist Makes a Home Visit
25. A Child Helps a Blind Man Cross a Street
26. White Cane Traveler
28. *Acknowledgements*
29. *Special thanks*

## While Waiting for the Ophthalmologist's Prognosis

The brain holds to
what little light remains
the chart's big E liminal
a moon with teeth tipped
in starless oblivion
20 over nearly nothing.

To measure is to hope
the everyday puzzle may be
more easily solved:
the coffee in the mug,
the salmon striped oxford,
in search of the right khakis,
the gas bill's opaque window.

Innumerable suns have been lost
in the iris, then refracted,
days settling like silt on the retina.

I think Giacometti,
hold steady one eye
an anesthetized target
ready for any clarity
of space and light
face framed bronze still.

Who wouldn't want to pull
any thread of color,
cobble together a Geneva street,
conjure angels ascending in marble?
I grip the exam chair's arms
and wait for the shadow to speak.

## Istanbul Busker

The young man plucks the gut strings
of an oud, flicks shrill runs
that swell in and out of reverberant cords
sullen as a hawker's calls for Turkish coffee.
There are no takers.

I stop sore tourist's feet
on my trek to the Bosporus
to listen, impossible not to soak
in his melody, a fringe
he sews to the afternoon's heavy drape.

*He is blind like you*
says a friendly German traveler
who shatters the privacy of shadow
cast by a hammam's brick facade
before the empty promenade.

It is an ocean
the busker and I both know,
no neat walls to shoreline or landmarks
to take us to familiar rooms,
only currents and faith
that crest and wane in slow decay
that trained fingers can only revive, the release
of our lives full of cautious steps.

## A Single Damn Word Never Finished

Was it for poetry I dangled
the weight of a braille typewriter?
For miles, I knew the map,
slumping homes, how to repair.

The carriage would not advance,
no expectation of leaving
one word for the next, no story
built of inconspicuous dots.

A fingertip skims, finds only the margin
a disconnected phone, burned linoleum,
a bottle's perfect mouth.

I touched a tuberculosis test card once
at seven, fascinated by the raised bump
that meant positive. My mother in
a vodka stupor tore it from me.

## Mainstream Test Case 1973

Dick and Jane waver
in my ten times magnifier,
letters like swimmers surface:
C's like sideways smiles,
J's like fish hooks,
G's like closed fists.

I practice the sounds
squint whole words into being
that blur back to the morning light
in Mrs. Byrd's first grade class.

I listened to twenty pencils scratch
in parallel lines of notebooks, tracks
I could not follow,
or believed I could not follow,
my nose tip graphite- gray from trying.

Where was my bus, I wondered,
the one that collected the county's special?

The shadows that appeared
on the playground
when I crossed the line into the normal
kids' space with the monkey bars
spawned faces, sunlit.
Were they smiling?

## Eminent Domain

One day I will tell you
why you stayed in the shadows
content to let the summer go
to voices not your own
played at thirty-three and a third RPMs.
How you waited through the slow grooves
for the needle's inevitable arc.

When the sheet doubled as a curtain
those mornings caught on nails.
The house's angles already condemned,
book-stacked stairs, broken floorboards heaving.
You baked on the apron porch, watched
the gray migrations of the days,
yourself a city in decline.

## SM Origin Story

Over donuts and bottomless coffee
the lighter of your eyes flicked—
our future, sugar, smoke. We tried
on dreams we thought were dreams.
The two mile walk to your back deck
the sum of our Catholic educations.
I folded my shame.
Your battle ax earrings swung.
And we jumped as friends,
breaking the water's skin
inviting in the stars. You held
me under the shimmer
for minutes. Feeling the slow burn,
I let my air go.

## Slow Night

The hearse's black mouth
spit out a father, my brother's father,
the man who raised me too, dead
from an agent orange and pneumonia cocktail.
December snow softened our thinning hair
as we cried at Taps, stood flag-straight for show.

Later, my brother kissed me—
full-lipped, a salivary misdemeanor
sloppy ring of our shared DNA
delivered in a Jameson whiskey vapor.
His cut chest and mechanic's guns
locked me in clumsy affection.
The vacuum tubes of his eyes
smoked hot, fired by hours
of playing his hollow-bodied guitar.

He hammered a dissident A chord
a fuzz cape he threw
over our shoulders, our blood
brought to the surface, fingertip blisters
popped, formed again, then popped.
Sliding down the guitar's neck to the G, the E,
we surrendered to the simple cord progression
I'd finally passed on.

## Drinking Alone

How calmly the cubes settle
in the tumbler
where twilight ambers.

The antidote to memory
lights the body's furnace,
tamps down the cold.

Once at a fetish street fair
a man-sized latex egg,
and in it, an alien.

The barrier of skin had dissolved.
A wet hand digs through
a breech to signal safe.

I take that hand in mine.

## How to Love a Mermaid

Replace reason with the green
swells of algorithms
churning to meet your rocky perch.

The possibility of a tail
scaled curves or eyes
urchin-colored, incalculable, awaits.

A chance crease in the current
may gesture you in.
Don't offer shells!

There will be time enough to build
an altar.  Don't offer birds
tiny lives that puzzle over

the silver hail of fish below.
A driftwood crown
will not woo her

to speak her name.
Gather mists to scale your skin instead.
Listen for gasps of waves.

Turn your back to the shore, the tongue
of smoke, uneven teeth of buildings—
the moon will choose you soon enough.

## Night Muse Gathers More Pulp for the Cosmic Pile

—opens me
like a letter,
lifts me
from sleep
with a red-nailed finger—
smooths me across the sky.

Night thinks
my news is nothing
if not quaint.
A few desperate lines
and she's got the story.
But my heart still pings
like an old Smith Corona.

## Snow Event

We believe the oracle for once,
the prophetic powers of doppler radar,
that the town will blaze white.

We set snow shovels as sentinels,
a salt offering, pairs of boots—
an altar at our door.

Our promised fate fills us as we strip
away the glaze of our routines.
We rub circles in glass to see out.

How easily the clean row of ranch homes
is negated, the greenery swallowed
in eddies and swirls of powder.

I see my childhood of escape
zipped up in a maroon striped snowsuit
buried beneath the frozen weight.

How good it was to be dead
for a time. The fortress lost and abandoned,
the calls of friends retreating.

Any blizzard will factor the neighborhood
sounds down to a distant whisper,
a prayer.

I know little of a mind of winter
only that the soft drifts will receive us
when we're ready to break their pristine white.

## Winter Ground

An apricot plucked
through a leafy sheath.

The effort rewarded
when you slip beneath the blanket's weight

fit your belly into the garden
hollow of my back, the single

candle holding out for sleep.
Did Plato really believe the gods

cleaved the mortal "one" in two?
I imagine our shadows are larger than two.

It's in these moments I want to tangle
the bones of our days and go

the way of the winter ground
to a memory of spring

clinging to you, to me, to our halves
of the seed, tightest at the day's end.

## Quarantine Window

Mud of cold coffee, low tide
in the cove. Clouds clear morning throats, spit drops staccato
prayer against our kitchen pane.

Another nest is slowly built
of forks and knives, cups parked
in the sink. Hours quantified:
the newly infected, the hospitalizations,
the ones who have died alone.

We eat more greens.
Take more vitamins.
Our hair grows wild.

We leave our pajamas on for work,
grateful to be avatars, squares
barely noticed in a grid
dissolving in the evening light.

## Glottal Stops

Birds dawdle before the day's heat
claws the courtyard's pomelo tree,
a pacific swallow, olive-backed sunbird, a zebra dove
light at my open window.

Corrugated steel peeks, adobe
brick walls, razor wire,
glass shards guard against the desperate
corner, children who thrust scentless sampaguitas
and bottled waters at slow walkers.

My thick tongue settles
complacent in its slick bed.
Puffs and rumbles of air and sound
rise as wind through stiff curtains.

I imagine you forming sounds
the duty of an eldest daughter
reeled back home to save a parent
to pack words into speeding hours as if
to avert your father's final breaths.

I practice cutting off the air
releasing it into the nose
and forward through the lips—
A, E, I, O, U.
I want to get this right
to climb into your sentences.

Smiling goes a long way
at the table: pancit, chicken adobo, and Lapu-Lapu
named after the chieftain who took down Magellan.
Our plates' topographies are marked by mountains
of food. I alone pile entrees on rice.

The motorcycle's sidecar contorts you.
I sit side-saddle behind the driver.
The wind absorbs my practice
of the passing street names, the scroll of eatery signs,
late night electric with families.
It will not slow down.

# Postcolonial Island Hopping

1.
Uniform vendors spirit passed
murmur the honorific mash-up
*maam-Sir, maam-Sir, maam-sir,*
*and peddle p*earls, pedicures, boiled peanuts.
We cling, their hot market
to the palms' splintered shadows.

2.
A coconut trunk bends low
to the white sand—
its marketing genius!
a deviation standing
among the picturesque.
Eager Instagrammers inch along
waiting for vacation shots
hands in a heart shape.

3.
A mango cheek.
Cheese-glazed sweet rolls.
Grit in the teeth.
A street cat named Putol
which means broken.

4.
Wrist bands admit us
to the tribe, glitter-painted.
Stage dancers dip and kick
jazz-hand salutes to the new moon.
We revel, too,
kick off our Crocs
to toe cool sand,
sink into our soles.

5.
Green swells
push and let go.
My body,
arms out,
legs stiff,
salt lips licked,
a timber adrift.

6.
The jungle comes fast
for slapped-up concrete walls,
glassless windows and verandas
split like fungused toenails.
A beachfront land-grab
gone belly up.

7.
The surf's rip and toe
sucks and heaves oily bile,
roars at the battered reef.
Rain of shells, wind dance, sand blow
night from above
touches night below.

8.
Neon spills blue chalk
on the night sand. Squid
boats burn at the horizon.
A name is nothing
to dance club subwoofers
and the wind.

9.
A dog mouths its own leash
pads alone along the boardwalk.
I make way for its belonging.

## Lady Liberty Begins to Fidget

She floats draped in metallic fabric
for slow hours, fixing her patinated copper crown.
Majestic by only a tourist's reckoning.

The matchstick- headed children who burn free
from their parents shriek toward her
on April's first hot day,

reach for her faux torch,
and guilt their parents into selfies
that go for five dollars each.

She grips their bills with a time-lapse sweep
of her free hand,
thinking how she'd like

to be less of a statue
one day, like the ladies
who claimed their evening benches,

money made and husbands buried,
they wrinkle smiles
at the democracy of squirrels
who fight over scraps in the grass.

## Public Art

I learn to live with his stare,
his weathered shovel face, the radiator belly,
the angler bolted outside my kitchen window
by the city's arts council.
His barbed wire net is cast for the season,
the artist's question drawn out like an accordion.
How he will bait the sandaled summer tourists
to chew on his symbolism, spit out
the surprise of his price tag.
His work is a snaggy conversation
he will keep to himself,
here where the tide of stroller drive-bys,
joggers, and paddle-borders drifts
eager for the cove's warming trend.
What days of boredom await him?

How he will enter their selfies
a mummer in a theater.
Only he and I will count
the horseshoe crabs' sudden die off.

## The Propellers

—sun their mangled and salt-stained wings
tarnished angels in every size
on the machine shop's sidewalk
a summer of miscalculations
waiting for a blunt fix.
The hammer lifts and strikes
lifts and strikes,
dissident grey detonations that bang
and decay down the row
of newly renovated three-deckers.
The neighborhood just wants to sleep,
turnover in high-thread-count sheets.
*Nobody is going anywhere today*
thinks the pock-faced man who hefts the hammer,
his ten-hour-days someone else's penance:
not the doctor with the lobster monger
side gig who cannot reach his traps,
not the yacht's preppy captain
who squints and twists his cap,
not even the sunset booze cruisers.
I count the ticks between the blows
wait for the next steel crash
that will rattle my morning, bleed
into my waking like the silted glass
of the tide's return.

## At the Canyon

the photo would have been morning perfect
at the canyon's lookout

squinted to a wafer
in the newlywed husband's viewfinder

his partner in pre-smile
selfie pose yet to be

struck like god and goddess
an instant both thought

would hover one day
in their smartphones

palmed in hands over cafe lattes
in morning's aging light

proof of that day at the lookout
of eternity, but for

the wind's capricious hand!
and now they tumble, vitriol grains

down to the chasm's scrub green floor
ballooning blue windbreakers

poor substitutes for wings,
a timeline jackpot

for thousands of eyes, dulled, now open
by light emitting diodes, living

their own sudden falls
in waking hands

a perfect tragedy
in which to believe.

## The Day I Deleted My Fitness App

Someone else can close
the open ring of their longing,
believe all they need is an encouraging blip
on days the gray washes in and settles.
I can't make the bed I lie in,
bring myself to remember the body.
Let me lengthen into the sun on my own.
That old jay still works
the squeaky gate hinge,
holds space in the garden
for the lilac's return.

## A Vision Rehab Therapist Makes a Home Visit

She cannot live with this loss
her retinas crimped and blotched like wet tissue
flowers once shaped for a rainy homecoming.
Her wallpaper stripes wriggle like snakes.
Her newspaper swims with insect rows.
Somewhere out there her unused car drifts.

We have all afternoon. I listen
in her kitchen, her pride silted over,
too early to teach her a new way to breathe,
the apparatus of blind living, my respirator,
just good enough for both of us.

Memories surface, silver in the light:
her penmanship's floweret loops,
a career of balancing books,
her husband's guiding hand.
We hold to each before it sinks
down to grief on the rickety table
among the stacks of unopened mail.

## A Child Helps a Blind Man Cross a Street

A tiny hand laid at my elbow
startles me— a child sent
from nowhere—her gentle pressure
ignores my impulse to pull free.
I could be anything to her:
a silver-maned blue horse that needs steadying,
a sluggish green dragon on a good day,
the neighborhood man who cannot see.

It is my wonder I put away
and a lesson for her
I grasp, my cane
two-touching our quiet street.
And because there is no danger
and because there is danger,
I give into her lead,
a parent's lesson she has received:
to do kindness. She has listened
and so I too listen
to her shy *you're welcome* after my thanks,
to the horizon's wash of distant cars.

## White Cane Traveler

Take a right at the worn clapboards.
Your palm finds the crease it knows.
Gather up a summer of dust,
haptic chatter with the afternoon.
Recall steps paced with breaths.
A picket fence becomes your guide,
bowed staves, musty sweet
pass you to the buckled street—
to stink weed in the sidewalks split,
the pithy prick of a rose tendril,
papery licks of hydrangea leaves,
the exhaling of the linden's hill.
Surrender to the slope ahead
where houses stagger, catch their step,
where wet paint scents the rooted path,
and hostas smother the corner green.
Turn here at the dogwood's end
to brush along wrought iron spines,
flecked and bent in unkept surrender,
drawing you down a crooked line
to church yard mums which suffocate.
The gritty hour's caught in the throat.
Broken stones stump your feet
and juniper bristles sprawl and reach.
Map again this tapestry
followed with a sensuous pace.
Map again this tapestry,
Tap step. Tap step.    Tap.

## Acknowledgements

Grateful acknowledgement is made to the editors of the journals in which these poems first appeared, in some cases in another form or under another title:

"How to Love a Mermaid" in *Bird Song Journal*

"At the Canyon" in *Boston Literary Journal*

"Night Muse Gathers More Pulp for the Cosmic Pile" in *Molecule*

"Quarantined Window" in *Voices Amidst the Virus* by Lily Poetry Review Books

"SM Origin Story" in *Of Rust and Glass*

"While Waiting for the Ophthalmologist's Prognosis" and "A Single Damn Word Never Finished" in *Disability: Visible and Invisible* by The Fourth River

"White Cane Traveler" in *The Saranac Review*

"Snow Event" in *The Ulu Review*

"Drinking Alone" in *The Whisky Blot*

"Lady Liberty Begins to Fidget" in *The Muddy River Poetry Review*

## Special Thanks

It is with deep and lasting gratitude that I thank the following persons for their continuing support, which has sustained me through the process of giving life to these poems and bringing this manuscript to its final form:

To Lily Poetry editors Eileen Cleary and Christine Jones, for taking me in and reviewing my poems with both warm applause and critical rigor.

To poets Tom Daley and Kevin McLellan, for inviting me into their workshops, which have given me community and pushed me to grow as a poet.

To photographer, Debi Milligan, for her stunning cover photo and portrait magic.

To poet Jennifer Martelli and again Tom Daley, for their generous blurbs.

To film maker and friend, Gina Kamentsky, whose discussions about the daily work of creating encouraged me through my unproductive stretches.

To poet and friend, Suzanne Mercury, just for being there.

And to my sweet life partner, Aurora Bautista, for her editing eye, listening ear, and serene, nourishing spirit.

## About the Author

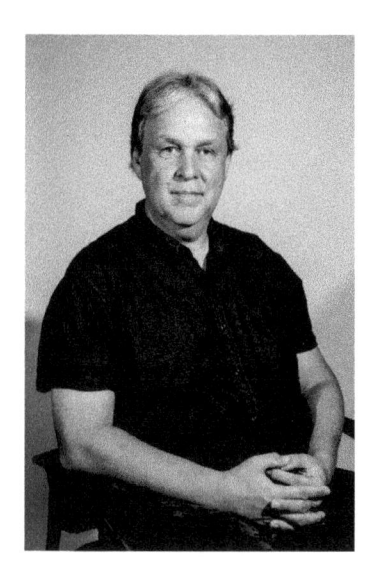

Darren Black's work has appeared in the *Muddy River Poetry Review, The Saranac Review online, Of Rust and Glass,* and in *Lily Poetry Review*'s anthology *Voices Amidst the Virus. Of Cautious Steps* is his first poetry collection. He lives on Massachusetts' north shore with his life partner and has recently retired from a rehabilitation counseling career. Darren, he/him, loves reading at local open mikes, playing music, connecting with new friends and places through travel, coaching adaptive sports, advocating for disability accommodations, and teaching others about blindness through his own experiences.

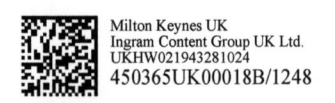